Recipes For Disease

Recipes For Disease

Book 1: Initial Findings

JP Grund

Library of Congress Control Number: 2008902532
ISBN: Hardcover   978-1-4363-3023-7
                      Softcover   978-1-4363-3022-0

This book was printed in the United States of America.

To order additional copies of this book, contact:
Xlibris Corporation
1-888-795-4274
www.Xlibris.com
Orders@Xlibris.com
48901

Contents

Introduction

My name is JP Grund. I've been training people in gyms since 1978. I have had hands-on experience with a vast array of ailments including, but not limited to, weight-loss, post-rehab, post-surgery, post-natal, anorexia, bulimia, OCD, COPD, AIDS, cancer of all kinds, schizophrenia, paranoia, arthritis, gout, etc. by providing exercise prescriptions to clients with specific needs. In my experience, I had always noticed a relationship between blood-type, diet and exercise, but I never had the lab, supplies or time to do the research. Also, I never knew exactly where to start looking. Additionally, I had never recommended any formal diet to my clients because they were always based on client testimonial and almost never based on any blood chemistry. Until I found the book "Eat Right for Your Type" by Dr. Peter J. D'Adamo.

The book gave me the blueprint I needed to put together all the information I had accumulated over a quarter-century and to correlate new information. The results have been astounding. I have found the book to be right on target for health, which is rare. Most of the formal diets on the market advertise short-term weight loss so the client can fit into that wedding dress or make an appearance at the up-coming high school reunion or the bathing suit season, etc., etc. That kind of diet is highly detrimental to the body and exists only to serve itself when the client returns the following season 25% heavier from lack of exercise and proper diet after quitting once the target weight was reached and the bathing suit fit to satisfaction. Disgusting and repetitive.

In "Eat Right For Your Type", foods are listed as beneficial (foods that act like medicines), neutral (foods that act like foods) and avoids (foods that act like poisons). The blood types used for this diet differ only by the antigen, the white blood cell, and not the red blood cell. The white blood cell differs only by the sugars on the antennae; O's have the basic type, fucose; A's have fucose plus the sugar N-acetyl-galactosamine; B's have fucose plus the sugar D-galactosamine; and AB's have the A-sugar and the B-sugar. Dr. D'Adamo gives a wonderful explanation of it in his book "Eat Right For Your Type".

The red blood cell is just a mechanism to transport nutrients and waste in and out of the body. It's the white blood cell, the antigen, that has to identify pathogens, contaminants and damaged or improper cells and then determine how to rid the body of them keeping away from healthy cells at the same time; it's the real thinking workhorse of the blood. Therefore, there are only four to be considered: A, O, B and AB. Statistically, A's, O's and B's comprise 97% of the population, so for the purposes of this book, AB's have been mostly ignored simply due to their availability. I intend to have more with subsequent books.

I decided to use myself as a guinea pig by being the personal trainer and staying in the beneficial foods as much as I could. To be brief, in the first twenty-four hours, all of my cravings disappeared and have never returned. That was July, 2005, and just the tip of the tip of the iceberg. I've been keeping a diary of my results. People started to see the changes that occurred with my body during the first week of the B-Type diet, which was a complete surprise. They started the diet. The results are like nothing I've ever seen. It's been so astounding that I donated the majority of my training-time to research. I am currently correlating diet, exercise, disease, family disease history and blood type.

I need more data to populate my database. I can't draw many conclusions without much more information. There are probably many more anomalies waiting to be discovered that we don't even know exist yet.

I want to make sure that the reader understands that nothing is 100%. All of these findings concern trends that comprise the majority, the vast majority or a despairingly different set of numbers that are unusual or out of the ordinary. There are known contradictions to certain trends that are usually avenues of new discoveries that generally open reasons for the preceding question, and/or basis for the trend, while rendering new questions at the same time. These are the paths of discovery.

I'm in need of blind demographics to fulfill research having to do with blood-type diets and their corresponding diseases. The trends that I have already uncovered are unusual, striking and very interesting. Some quick conclusions have been found, such as

—People with A-type blood who eat meat have high cholesterol.

—People with O-type blood who do not eat meat are anemic.

—A beneficial food for an A does as much good as an avoid food for an O does bad.

—I.T. departments have a despairingly large percentage of B-types.

Here are some of the trends / areas of study currently being conducted:

1. Gestational Blood Types

2. Eating Disorder patients, Alcoholics and Obsessive compulsions

3. Romantic Compatibilities

4. The Pathology Of Diabetes

5. The Pathology Of Idiocy

6. Addison's disease in A-type blood and its connection to heartburn

7. Prostate cancer in B-type blood

8. Pathology of Diabetes

9. High cholesterol in O's & Anemia in A's

10. Pork's relationship to tumors

11. Scarring of the body

12. The neurology of B's

13. Longevity, especially in A's

14. Immature palette

Each of these trends, or areas of study, has real data to back them up, so far, and I have included a portion of the blind data. I'd like to disprove what I can, but I need much more information to prove or disprove any trends that appear. The following is a list of the fields of information in the blind demographics.

1. Gender

2. Year Of Birth

3. Blood Type

4. Ailments and/or Current Prescriptions

5. Mother's Blood Type

6. Blood Type of Spouse or significant other

7. Staple Diet

8. Contact info (if applicable)

Scarring Of The Body

Scarring of the body is really nothing more than aging. Sometimes it happens faster than other times. Scarring, or aging for that matter, is damage to the body that is irreversible, without some sort of stem cell replacement application which appears to be years down the road.

A good example of scarring of the body is diabetes. Basically, once the pancreas is damaged to the point of insufficient insulin production, it has been scarred. Nothing short of stem cells will rectify the situation. It could be said the diabetic pancreas has aged well beyond its years.

Surgeries are good examples of quick scarring of the body. I've seen countless patients over the years who would go through surgery and wonder why they had so much scar tissue build up causing them to not function properly after recovery, while all the time they were eating wrong for their blood-types; mostly pork. Then I've seen the patients over the years who would just happen to eat right for their blood-types after surgery and recover quickly with little scar tissue. At the time, nothing was known about blood-type diets, so the doctors would just shrug their shoulders and lump it all on the most convenient scapegoat of them all: genetics. Doctors have genetics and meteorologists have the weather; they still get paid regardless of success.

The slowest scarring of the body is aging. The body's ability to exactly replicate dying or damaged cells is never 100% and can only be maximized by giving the body what it needs to rebuild. If the digestion can't process it or if the blood can't transport it, the body can't use it. It's as simple as that.

The O-Cycle

I've long since noticed a trend in people with O-type blood that I'll call the O-Cycle. The typical O wakes up in the morning and can't start until that first cup of coffee. Without the coffee, the person is not fit to be around. The typical O may drink as few as one cup of coffee to drinking all the way throughout the day.

Regardless, by the time the O goes to bed at night, sleep becomes difficult due to the caffeine intake throughout the day. The typical O goes to the bedtime kitchen and generally finds some sort of dairy product to go to sleep. You wouldn't believe how many O's have told me they eat ice cream to get to sleep. Being an extreme avoid for people with O-type blood, dairy products digest poorly and slow the entire digestive tract and overall metabolism. By morning, the O wakes groggy, sluggish and ill-tempered; until the first cup of coffee. And the cycle continues day in and day out.

The list of diseases and illnesses that are created from this O-cycle are so numerous, they range from weight-gain and allergies to colon issues and early menopause; and everything in between. There are truly too many possibilities as a direct result of the O-cycle to possibly list here in this book; it would be an encyclopedia. Why? Because the two culprits, caffeine and lactose, are not only highly toxic to an O-type system, but tend to affect the O-type body in completely separate and unique ways.

Lactose is commonly referred to as 'milk sugar'. It's digested by an enzyme called lactase. Lactase is produced in the pancreas. Since O-type's evolved from the original blood-type who were carnivores, and hardly ever ate any sugar-type foods, their pancreases never had to digest anything like milk or any dairy product. Therefore, lactase production for an O is a Herculean task compared to a B, the dairy people, or even an A, for who dairy is an avoid as well. When an O-type ingests dairy, along with a poor O-type diet, a myriad of aliments, including diabetes, can be the result. This is a type of scarring of the body.

Caffeine in an O-type body causes the hormones to become unbalanced. This causes other organs to have to work harder to correct the situation. At first, the body is young and can accomplish this feat with little notice, but the strain on the overworked organs is insidious over the years and eventually the body begins to have difficulties producing enough hormones; namely estrogen. Before too long, the levels fall too far and symptoms of menopause begin to appear. This is a type of scarring of the body.

The necessity of the coffee and the quantity ingested appear to depend on other avoid foods being eaten throughout the day; namely, for example and among many other foods, corn products because of its inhibition of insulin production in people with O-type blood. One of the worst combinations is an O-type who drinks coffee and eats corn products. It is one of the worst and most prevalent recipes for disease, mainly because the prevalence of O-type people and such corn products as high fructose corn syrup, and all the other names it goes by.

In the past, I have had limited success with suggesting trying to replace coffee in the morning with Damiana due to its energy releasing properties and its relationship to balancing hormones for Menopause. This is mostly effective with women, however finding a substitute for men has proven to be a bit unique and proprietary to the patient; in that, they usually end up finding their own substitute, so far. This could be because coffee doesn't have the extreme effects on male hormones the way it does to female hormones, solely because women have all the chemistry to balance in the first place and therefore they have more to disturb. Men may find it easier to substitute naturally. Instead, the male O who drinks coffee finds digestive issues that accumulate over the years to affect the colon adversely. Replacing dairy at night to go to sleep appears to be more difficult for O-type men than it does for O-type women. That being said, I may be splitting hairs. It's difficult for either. The substitutes over the years have ranged from Melotonin to Valerian root and as extreme as Marijuana. Sleep inducers are varied and many.

It appears that exercise is the best substitute for coffee and dairy for the O. Sorry.

Are there sleep inducers and energy releasers more blood-type compliant? Can the entire over-the-counter industry be revamped to be blood-type compliant?

Gestational Blood Types

For our purposes, the term 'gestational blood-type' refers to the mother's blood type and the child's blood type. The mitochondrial DNA passed solely from the mother tends to pass traits of the mother.

For example, an O-type who is born of a mother with a non-gestational blood type, that is a blood type that is different from the fetus, will exhibit traits similar to the mother's blood type. Similarly, an O-type, born of an O-type mother, exhibits extreme O-type characteristics. I have found an A-type, born of an O-type mother, who is able to follow her body's call for the beneficial A-type diet just like an O-type person does normally. I have found a B-type, born of an O-type mother, who seems to derive more beneficial effects from red meats than a normal B-type and has more stomach acid than a normal B-type.

At first, it appeared there were to be sixteen different sub-types to homo sapien and I constructed the diagram below (4 X 4). Each number refers to a corresponding explanation below; not all are filled in because I need more information. However, I may have been premature. Read the chart and their corresponding explanations and I 'll continue telling of where this trend is going awry.

		Your	Mother's	Blood	Type
		A	B	O	AB
Your	A	1	2	3	4
Blood	B	5	6	7	8
Type	O	9	10	11	12
	AB	13	14	15	16

1. Known as the straight-A, the A-type whose mother was an A also usually exhibits extreme A-type blood tendencies. These include a diet that is not in the beneficial for A-type blood and can be in the avoid foods for A-type blood for the vast majority of their diet. They tend to eat poorly

for A-type blood and generally can't read what their bodies are telling them they need to eat.

3. A person with A-type blood whose mother had O-type blood generally can read what their body wants to eat. As a result, they are eating a surprising amount of beneficial foods for A-type blood all on their own and only by listening to their body's call for food. This is unusual for people with A-type blood and is more normal for people with O-type blood.

6. Known as the straight-B, the B-type whose mother was a B also usually exhibits an uncanny nutrient reserve. These people tend to go without breakfast and yet have no discernable sugar-low.

7. A person with B-type blood whose mother had O-type blood generally exhibits a higher stomach acid content than a normal B-type. High stomach acid content is generally associated with people with O-type blood. As a result, some neutral meats for B-types may be more beneficial than with a normal B-type person. Bison and steak could give better results than a straight B-type person. Also, dairy intake, though still normally massive for a B-type, has its limits. Lactase can become depleted if an extreme amount of lactose is ingested at once. Ice cream seems to be a worse avoid food than the normal B-type. Pancreatic issues can become apparent if alcohol and poor diet are regular, which is a trait of people with O-type blood.

11. Known as the straight-O, an O-type person with an O-type mother will have extreme O-type tendencies. They show signs of an extremely weak pancreas to the point of diabetes, pancreatitis and liver issues. They have low blood sugar issues indicative of a sluggish pancreas. This results in mood swings and unclear thought. Their high stomach acid content can easily produce ulcers with a poor diet and/or alcohol.

Where has it gone awry? In number 11, the straight-O, I may have found two different types. There appears to be one type of straight-O that is prone to diabetes and another that is prone to arthritis. Additionally, it appears the two don't mingle; that is, the straight-O either gets arthritis or diabetes. I can't seem to find one that has both, but I need more data.

The book tells of one of the first adverse agglutinations they found in the lab, which was with O-type blood. White potatoes are listed as an avoid food for O's because they found that it agglutinates improperly in O-type blood and piles up in the joints as arthritis. I have seen this to be true throughout the data and the years.

This sub-type that appears to have gone awry is significant because both diabetes and potatoes are sugar related. Additionally, over the years I have noticed that, comparatively speaking, O's tend to have weaker pancreases than the other blood types. This would make sense on an anthropological basis. After all, the O was the original blood type back when mankind was eating nothing but meat and had no sugars, complex or simple, in their diets whatsoever; the O didn't need a heavy-duty pancreas to process sugars because they never ate any.

Therefore, it would make sense that, instead of gestational blood type trends following solely the antigen, it could be said that it is much more genetic than that and it actually follows genetics down to the red blood cell. Therefore, there would be sixty-four different subtypes (8 X 8) of homo sapiens.

Where this portion of the research could send us is so unpredictable, I feel I have opened a door to an area so vast and dark that it will take a long time to harvest all the results from all the information. The possibilities are endless and very exciting, but I need much more information.

Eating Disorder Patients, Alcoholics and Obsessive Compulsions

I have found a trend in eating disorder patients. Starting with O-Type blood, during their worst years of their ED (Eating Disorder), they ate 100% avoid foods for their O-type blood. Contrarily, I have found that normal O-type people tend to hit their prescribed O-type beneficial diet naturally and on their own without knowing anything about the book.

Paradoxically, I have found ED patients with A-type blood ate virtually 100% beneficial during their worst years of their ED, whereas I have found normal people with A-type blood eat avoid foods for A-type blood on a very regular basis.

It could be said that normal A's and O's miss and hit their respective beneficial foods because of society being so carnivorous, which hits for O's and misses for A's. However, it begs the question of what is going on with ED patients. It would appear they have a natural mental craving that is different from their normal counterparts.

Furthermore, the trend appears to surround around the patient's intake of whole wheat and appears to be related to alcoholism as well. I have found that when alcoholics and ED patients get away from whole wheat and stay with sprouted wheat breads, their cravings and overall thought processes change for the better. It appears the thought of drinking or acting out their ED cravings never seem to enter the mind. It's almost as if it never gets to the conscience thought process and never even gets a chance to become a craving.

The theory is that since the brain works solely on simple sugars, the starchy carbs that the simple sugars come from could carry with them characteristics particular to the starchy carb source of the simple sugar, which could play a significant role as to their effect on the brain.

Brenda (not real name) was quite the specimen. She still stays in touch and the updates are worthy of the end of a huge novel; easily too long to tell here. There was a number of very interesting things that came out of the Brenda experience. One of them was the connection between the source of metabolized sugar and the reaction in the brain. I found that her obsessive tendencies subsided significantly and quickly when she switched to a sprouted wheat source of bread, namely Ezekiel bread. I have found another diabetic-prone teen has better attention span and less frustration with learning when he stays away from whole wheat products, eats Ezekiel bread and keeps his blood sugar level even. Both are O-types and therefore have a very narrow window of breads that are not to be avoided by them; O's and breads don't get along. The book, *Eat Right For Your Type*, explains the antigen/lectin connection and how the lectins are destroyed when the seed covering is destroyed when wheat sprouts; whole wheat is a very bad thing.

My hypothesis is the source of the metabolized sugar on which the brain runs and operates is of a very significant value. It's like an engine that runs on either low-octane fuel or high-octane fuel; it simply runs better on the higher octane, but runs OK on the low-octane. In the brain, the different reactions to different sugars appear to be wide and very significant.

Specifically, as in OCD patients, the chemicals in the neuron that fail to jump across and stay on the other side of the neuron, thus failing to turn on that neuron, do so possibly because the simple sugar that runs that neuron is a poor match for that blood-type. The simple sugar either was processed improperly or carried a poor characteristic with it from the starchy carbohydrate from which it was made. Something along the line of the difference between super unleaded and regular unleaded in your car; one tends to run better than the other. Does this trend remain constant over the general populous? Does it appear to be a possible therapy? Is there a cure?

As with everything else in this study, I need much more information. One possible result from this particular section of the study is that it may produce a treatment for crystal meth addiction. Crystal Meth in a capsule taken on a full stomach while limiting breads to only Ezekiel and/or Manna (Essene) bread could be the combination that gives the addicts a viable option other than 'cold-turkey', which can be too much for an addict to take. The oral intake of crystal meth reduces the physical punch the drug gives the addict, while the mental addiction of snorting the drug or smoking the drug is replaced by a quick swallow of a capsule. As the addiction wanes, the dosage is gradually reduced until it's gone.

On a possibly related note, I've noticed a paradox between A's and O's. A beneficial for an A goes a long way and just as far as an avoid for an O. That is to say that A's derive as much good from a beneficial as O's derive bad from an avoid. It seems A's can survive a torrent of avoids and save themselves with small amounts of beneficials, whereas O's tend to stay in the beneficials naturally and every little avoid for them is associated with some disorder. Why?

Romantic Compatibilities

In my research, I started to notice that married couples who had been married for decades had a high percentage of common blood types; that is, they were pairs of the same blood types whether it be a pair of O's or a pair of A's, or a pair of B's. I don't have enough AB's in my data to establish a trend, yet. I was finding that these matching pairs were the couples who were together decades and lived happily ever after.

I started to theorize that it had to have something to do with moods and mood swings. If it was daily moods and mood swings that determined marital longevity, then it would follow that glucose would be key. After all, the brain runs on sugar. Therefore, the couple's common beneficial meats would supply the protein necessary to regulate glucose absorption into the blood. If the husband has the same glucose reaction to the foods he eats as does the wife, then they should have the same moods and mood swings simultaneously, as well as overall physical reactions to the same foods ingested.

So, I got to thinking that if this trend follows their meats they have in common, then O's and B's should be a pretty good match since they share beneficial and neutral meats such as lamb, mutton, venison and beef. I have found, in the numbers, that O's and B's do indeed have marital longevity. My parents, for example, were a B/O combination and they were happily married for fifty years till death did them part. It seems that B/O combinations have a slightly higher incidence of divorce than matching pairs, but they are still very compatible.

So, once again, I figured if this theory holds true, then O's and A's should be fairly toxic due to the fact that they have no common beneficial meats and the only common neutral meat they have is chicken. I found, in the data so far, that if an O/A combination survives divorce, then one or both of them are in very poor health due to eating for the other person. The vast majority end in divorce.

So, again, I postulated that B's and A's should be even more toxic than O's and A's because B's and A's share no common meats, whether beneficial or neutral; chicken is an extreme avoid for B's due to a powerful lectin found mostly in breast meat. I started looking for B and A romantic combinations. To my utter astonishment, I couldn't find the first pair in almost two and a half years of looking. I was shocked that it took so long. To date, I have only found three pairs of B/A combinations that are unconfirmed blood-types; they have not been tested. The only common trend in these three pairs is their education and overall intelligence; both husbands and wives are successful and very smart. This is one of the most striking parts of the blood type trend research. I need more data.

This romantic blood-type compatibility trend is not without its exception. I know of one couple who recently celebrated their fortieth wedding anniversary in 2006 with opposing blood types. She is an O and he is an A. These two are retired and have done everything from shopping at the grocery store together to going to the post office together from day one. They're inseparable. It's quite cute. You have to call over at their house before you visit just so you don't catch them having sex. All that being said, they do follow one ominous pattern: whenever there's an A and an O in a romantic relationship, one always suffers until that person gets away from that relationship. Generally, one is usually eating for the other one. In this case, the husband has always had the diseases down through the years. Sadly, these two are so much in love and do everything together, I fear that when one of them passes away, the other's body will have the potential to live for quite some time afterwards, but will die of loneliness. I hope not.

I'm always eager to disprove all these trends that materialize. I'm very eager to disprove this romantic compatibility trend, if possible. What if mankind's underlying reason for war and conflict throughout the centuries was because of incompatible blood types in combination with the foods being ingested? What if that's the underlying reason for criminal behavior?

The Pathology Of Diabetes

Possible Equation:
O-Type + Dairy + Corn + White potatoes - Fish = Diabetes

The pathology of diabetes starts with eating the wrong foods. Many of the foods in the avoids lists for their perspective blood types cause the body to do things that are sugar related. This should not be a surprise because the main job of the digestive system is to deliver and maintain proper blood-sugar levels. It seems blood-sugar levels are the essence of life. Many of these foods inhibit proper insulin production and/or metabolism, but the medical industry, even if the doctor goes that far, never say why.

Eating wrong foods for your blood-type can cause conditions such as hypothyroidism. Causing the overall metabolism to slow down, the body compensates by ever so lightly turning on the adrenals so a small amount of insulin, cortisol, etc. leaks into the blood like a leaky faucet. We'll call this phenomenon leaky adrenals.

Stress is probably the biggest cause of leaky adrenals. The worker is at work all day long suppressing leaky adrenals that occur with every paper cut, bad customer service experience, poor driving experience to work and on the way home, etc, etc., etc.

Pre-historic man would burn off those adrenals by chasing down a lonely buffalo, beating the crap out of it and slaughtering it in the open field to feed the group. He would then burn off the resulting fat and cholesterol by chasing down the next large prey to eat.

Modern men don't chase buffalo's or any other beast to kill it and eat it. Instead, we go to the grocery store and buy something already processed. We go home, cook it and eat it. The leaky adrenals never get burned and, instead, they are chemically metabolized by insulin produced in the pancreas. Thus, the pancreas stays slightly turned on and working virtually constantly producing what the medical industry has long since found to be a 'sluggish pancreas' due to the fact the doctors see the resulting sugar-low known as hypoglycemia. The immunities eventually see that the pancreas is constantly putting out a quantity of insulin and, therefore, consider it a threat to the body's overall well-being. In an effort to protect the body, they start attacking the insulin islets in what has become to be known as an 'autoimmune reaction'. Eventually, after years of this process going unchecked, the pancreas can no longer keep up the production of insulin while being attacked by auto immunities, so it burns out and diabetes results.

On top of that, the pancreas has had to produce digestive enzymes, such as lactase and amylase, all those years for a person who eats the wrong thing, thus, placing even more long-term stress on the pancreas which is already working to produce a steady flow of insulin to counteract leaky adrenals.

It should be no surprise how prevalent diabetes is in the US.

Lack of exercise causes the adrenal fluids to be metabolized almost entirely by the pancreas with its slow production of insulin which metabolizes the resulting sugar in the blood put there by the leaky adrenals.

When consistent daily exercise is performed, the slightly elevated blood-sugar is metabolized by physical action rather than chemically by pancreas-produced insulin. Thus, the pancreas can rest, if it's fully grown, or grow, if it's immature.

Are O's more susceptible to leaky adrenals due to their carnivorous nature? Are they more susceptible to stress? Can prescriptions and even synthetic insulin be produced more compliant with the patient's blood-type? Can all medications, surgeries, anesthesias and every aspect of the medical community be tailored for specific blood-groups? Is this why doctors currently get different results for two separate patients when both patients have the same ailments, physical parameters and prescriptions?

The Pathology of Idiocy

The following example demonstrates the pathology of idiocy best.

The Teacher always saw the student's mother have sugar-lows in her blood and the Teacher always told her she was a candidate for diabetes. Her sugar-lows were so pronounced, it was very easy to see what was happening.

Her self induced stress always was a factor. The self-induced stress she generated would cause the adrenals to 'leak'. Her slow reacting pancreas would turn on late and would not stop producing insulin causing her blood sugar to hit lows and wreak havoc on her system with mood swings, weight loss and incoherent thought processes.

Combine that with the constant ingestion of milk into an O-type diet and she ultimately became diabetic due to burning out a pancreas that never had the chance to turn off due to self induced stress and a very bad O-type diet.

The student is an O-type with the exact same metabolism as his mother. When the Teacher started home schooling the student in eighth grade, his sluggish pancreas would cause a sugar-low by 10am at the latest. The brain, running on specific sugars metabolized in the body, is the first organ to turn off and therefore, he stopped learning. It was like teaching a rock. The sugar-low switch was just as pronounced and easily recognizable as his mother's. The first day in home schooling before 10am when the hunger hit, he said, "It's OK, I can keep going. I have to do it everyday in government school."

A small nuclear bell went off in the Teacher's head. No wonder the student was learning very little in government school. In government school, he would have to go from approximately 10am to after noon on a severe sugar-low with the learning part of the brain turned off. Even if he got nutrition at that point, it was too late. If the brain runs on low fuel for too long, it will tire easily and will need not only nutrition, but sleep as well. Therefore, after lunch, at government school, came the inevitable sleepiness and the rest of the day was wasted. This would happen on a daily basis.

The teacher, at 10am rather than after noon, told him to eat. He ate, his brain turned back on and he continued to learn.

He fought the sugar-low at first. The next day he tried to hide it, but it was so pronounced and easily recognizable that it's just like turning off the brain switch. The Teacher told him he was hungry, but he said he wasn't and he could continue. He was told to just stand up and he'd be hungry. He got up from his chair and made it only to the doorway before he said, "OK, I'm hungry. I can eat." He ate, his brain turned back on and he continued learning.

After that, he ate when he felt it and he has become very knowledgeable in the O-type diet. He then did in school in an hour what use to take him two weeks to do.

This is why his mother never graduated high school. She has the exact same metabolism as the student, but when she was in middle school during puberty when these huge sugar-lows were being produced by a sluggish pancreas, she had no one to home school her and therefore never developed her brain. It simply shutdown during school, didn't get exercised and never developed. It's all really quite simple.

This is The Pathology of Idiocy. A middle school student enters middle school just at the same time the hormones are making the brain grow in its pubescent growth spurt; the brain's largest growth spurt in the student's life and the second since the "terrible two's". The fuel for the brain is pure sugar, so when the student's glucose level in the blood hits that low blood-sugar level, the first thing the body turns off are the organs that use sugar heavily. Since the brain is the heaviest user, especially when the student is trying to learn and grow at the same time, the body turns it off first. The student sits in the classroom not learning or exercising a growing brain that depends on exercise to develop properly during the growth years. By the time the student enters high school, the student possesses a woefully underdeveloped brain that is then considered post-pubescent, adolescent and almost adult-sized. There won't be another growth spurt in the student's life that will rectify what went underdeveloped during the middle school years. The student moves forward into adult life struggling to make things go right day-to-day and never coming close to any leap of intelligence.

Now, multiply that by an entire nation, then multiply that by the past 30 years and the product becomes 21st century America: an adult-aged child-like society that mortgages for fun, saves very little and lives paycheck-to-paycheck. It's a 'Twilight Zone' society that can't even begin to make a thoroughly logically based decision on the facts nor know when a decision can't be made due to lack of facts. They draw foregone conclusions processed haphazardly in brains that never got the chance to develop properly during the one time in their lives when it needed to grow and would never get the chance again. They repeatedly fill the ranks of the prescriptions for everything from antidepressants to cold remedies that do nothing but mask symptoms and never address the cause of the ailment without ever knowing any better.

America now has an intellectual malaise very similar to the intellectual malaise that seemed to permeate the beginning of the decline of The Roman Empire. There seems to be debate over exactly what caused the lack of intellect in Rome and its effects, but it was there, regardless, for about the first hundred years of the beginning of the decline of The Roman Empire. The meek have long since inherited this Earth.

Is this pathology of idiocy more prevalent in O's due to their carnivorous pancreas? Do some kids handle the glucose lows better than others? Why? How? Do they continue with good grades? Is it as simple as combining a proper protein and carbohydrate in the previous meal, such as breakfast? How does this relate to immature palette?

Addison's Disease In A-Type Blood

And Its Connection To Heartburn

Possible equation:
A-type + tomato products - fish - vegetables = Addison's Disease

The following is a working example of a health prescription written for a client I recently found who has Addison's disease and heartburn. Heartburn is very significant in a person with A-type blood due to the fact that A's generally possess an alkaline digestive system. An acidic condition in a person with A-type blood is worthy of a deeper look.

"Female, A-Type
Chronic Heartburn
Addison's Disease

The female, who is A-Type blood, born in 1977, has chronic heartburn to the point of having an ant-acid, such as Tums, on-hand at all times. This is rare because of the A's typically alkaline digestive juices. She was first diagnosed with Addison's Disease at age seven. Addison's disease is a hormone deficiency (not enough hormone) caused by damage to the outer layer of the adrenal gland (the part known as the adrenal cortex).

In the female's case, doctors have determined that her Addison's disease has been caused from the autoimmune disorder where the antigens attack the adrenal cortex. She has been off her medications for four years.

Her mother is an O-type, so her diet follows the natural callings of an A-type blood body. She doesn't eat a lot of red meat; it makes her nauseous. This is why her cholesterol is OK. However, that being said, her diet in twenty-four hours consisted of a slim-jim for breakfast, no lunch and a Coke and a fried, boneless chicken breast for dinner. Generally, she eats tomato products like they're going out of style, bread products, pasta, and vinegar. (She ingests no fish and little vegetables; both of which are essential to the A-type system.) It would be no surprise that this is exactly where her heartburn is coming from (if not the cause of the Addison's as well). If this diet continues, an ulcer, at the very least, will occur, if it hasn't already and then proceed to affect the colon; just the same way an O-type does to the colon after years of mismanaging acid. Additionally, Addison's will worsen and develop into any one, or combination, of the ailments associated with Addison's, which ultimately hastens an early demise.

The following is a health prescription based mainly on correcting immediate problems such as chronic heartburn and symptoms of Addison's disease such as lack of energy, which are the two sources of future health problems. Once these problems are eradicated, other problems should lessen or disappear. This prescription was derived by correlating information from two main sources. They are "Eat Right For Your Type" by Dr. Peter J. D'Adamo and "Prescription For Nutritional Healing" by Phyllis and James Balch. By correlating these two books along with my own experience, this prescription for health should show results quickly if followed precisely.

Keep in mind that your dietary list, according to "Eat Right For Your Type" by Dr. Peter J. D'Adamo, includes foods not only on the beneficial list, but also all the foods listed in the neutral lists as well. All you have to avoid are the foods on the avoid lists. Many people start to think they have nothing to eat, whereas, in reality, you have more variety with this diet than without. Just avoid the avoids and try to stick with the beneficials as much as you can.

The bad news first. Absolutely no beef products, no pork products, no whole wheat products, no tomato products, no dairy products, no milk, no ice cream, no potatoes, no olives, no peppers, no cabbage, no english muffins, no seeds, and no lima, garbanzo or kidney beans. No sodas, no artificial sweeteners, no alcohol, no shrimp, no flounder, no catfish, no clams, no lobster, no banana products, no licorice, no orange juice or orange products. If you take a diuretic, consult your doctor before supplementing with calcium and vitamin D.

The good news. You have three land animal protein sources that are neutral for A-type blood and serve as good protein sources, which are chicken, cornish hens and turkey. In moderation, eggs are a good source of protein if the cholesterol level is OK. Your beneficial (medicinal) protein sources are found almost exclusively in fish. Sardines are a highly beneficial and medicinal source of protein, soluble calcium and zinc and they reduce inflammation; they are also a cancer and diabetes superbeneficial for A's. Medicinal fish protein sources are numerous and varied. Some examples include monkfish, cod, grouper, rainbow trout, salmon, sardine, red snapper, etc.

Your varied amino acids are essential in combating cancer, depression and diseases such as diabetes. Eating a combination of meats, eggs and fish should supply a good array of amino acids. L-carnitine is an amino acid that is essential in promoting good circulation. However, red meats, which do not digest properly in the A-type alkaline digestive system and must be avoided, are the primary dietary source of L-carnitine. Other A-type animal-based foods containing L-carnitine include mackerel, salmon and turkey. Tempeh (fermented soybeans), sprouted wheat, and avocados also contain this nutrient. L-carnitine is available in synthetic form as a pill and/or capsule, but is not recommended since there are plenty of food sources.

Go to http://www.dadamo.com/typebase4/typeindexer.htm to see different foods and how they affect the body.

I cannot over-emphasize the benefits you, in particular, will derive from sushi. The sushi is dipped in soy sauce, which is not only a beneficial for A's, but it also has the salt content that you need due to the lowering levels of sodium caused by the Addison's condition. Additionally, sushi made with such beneficial fish as salmon has a large amount of fish oils (fats) that correct so many things such as chronic heartburn. Thirdly, the varied amino acid profiles derived from raw fish is exactly the recipe for longevity into triple digits for A's and one of the best ways to avoid cancer for A-type blood. Sushi is highly recommended due to the added tremendous benefits from not being cooked; the enzymes stay in tact when raw thus aiding in digestion and relieving some need for more acid in the stomach. Cooked is OK too, just remember that grilled or baked has less fat and cholesterol than fried.

There are other sources of protein for A's besides meats and fish. Snails, *helix pomatia*, agglutinate to two of the most common forms of breast cancer cells in A's and AB's. Peanuts are beneficial for A-type blood. Salted peanuts are especially good for you due to the low sodium condition caused by Addison's. Peanut butter is a beneficial source of protein for A's. Just remember to get the low fat peanut butter. A peanut butter and jelly sandwich is beneficial for A's when made with a beneficial jelly/preserve, such as plum, pineapple, blueberry, etc., and a beneficial bread, such as essene (manna) bread, rice cakes, soy flour bread or, though it's a neutral for A's, oat bread. Though the book, *Eat Right For Your Type,* says that peanuts are beneficial for A's, a person with a history of any colon disease, such as Crohn's disease, might be better suited to steer clear of the whole nut due to the possibility of developing diverticulitis, which can lead to colon cancer. You have no history, so it's something to keep in mind.

Zinc is important for anyone due to its effectiveness on immunities and depression. Zinc can be found in eggs, fish, poultry and zinc lozenges. It is easily lost due to colon conditions such as diarrhea.

The list of beneficial and neutral vegetables and fruits for A-type blood is so long, you'll simply have to go to the website and look whenever you're curious about a particular food. I'll list a few of the exceptional beneficials that tend to help in areas that are specific for you. By all means, remember there are many more options than what I'm mentioning here. You truly have a variety available in vegetables and fruits that is unparalleled in any other blood type.

Dandelion greens are not only a good source of zinc and calcium, but they also are considered highly beneficial for A's due to their balancing of certain chemicals in the blood, such as indican levels and/or polyamine synthesis. Seaweed contains vitamin D which is necessary for calcium absorption and has recently been found to have anti-cancer qualities. Oatmeal, broccoli and green leafy vegetables, such as collard greens and dandelion greens, are highly beneficial and medicinal sources of calcium. Oatmeal tends to boost immunities in A's. Since oranges are out of the picture for A's due to the acid, vitamin C can be found in grapefruit, which is also a cancer superbeneficial for A's. Grapefruit is considered highly beneficial and medicinal for A's due to its boosting of the immunities. Kiwi is a good source of vitamin C also. Pineapple helps to reduce inflammation. Pineapple boosts immunities and is a diabetes superbeneficial in A's. Additionally, pineapple contains an enzyme called bromelein which helps absorb calcium and digest protein. Eat a little pineapple at the end of each meal.

When it comes to bread, my experience could fill a book. The benefits of Ezekiel bread cannot be exaggerated, for all blood types. The problem is the taste. Therefore, a slice should be toasted and then a beneficial fruit preserve should be spread over the toasted slice and eaten as the dessert at the end of the meal. Pineapple, fig, blueberry and plum preserves are just a few suggestions that are all beneficial for A's. Once eaten, the body's call for dessert (sugar) is satisfied on a very healthy basis.

Soy milk is highly beneficial due to its boosting of immunities. It's a cancer and diabetes superbeneficial for A's. Soy milk has phytoestrogens that help hormone balance. The main reason for osteoporosis, bone loss, is hormonal imbalances generally caused by menopause and/or bad diet in conjunction with age. Get the vanilla or chocolate soy milk; the plain tastes really nasty.

Dairy can be tolerated in small amounts, but there are no dairy beneficials for A's. However, dairy should be avoided for weight-loss for A's and O's. I'll mention a few here, but the fewer you can do, the better. Yogurt is a neutral and a good source of calcium for A's. It provides good bacteria (acidophilus) for the lower colon thus correcting digestive problems and aiding in people prone to digestive ailments. Yogurt has optimal amino acid (lysine/arginine) ratio. Kefir is another dairy product that has the same characteristics as yogurt for A's. The key to enjoying things like kefir and yogurt is to get them with a beneficial fruit that you like. If you like pineapple, its benefits cannot be over emphasized. Peach kefir seems to be tasty. Pineapple yogurt is available, but a look at your beneficial fruit list in the book, "Eat Right For Your Type" by Dr. Peter J. D'Adamo, might give you some more ideas.

Onions and garlic are good sources of sulpher which the body needs to absorb calcium for all blood types. Onions and garlic are cancer superbeneficials for A's and are considered highly beneficial due to their medicinal properties that boost your immunities.

Coffee is listed as a beneficial for A's due to its immunity building properties and increased stomach acid. However, your chronic heartburn would tend to move coffee into more of an avoid than it would be in neutral or beneficial. Caffeine can have an adverse effect on calcium absorption, but it seems to be minimal if not non-existent in A's. Use de-caf in moderation only long after the heartburn has been corrected.

I have found incredible digestive results with drinking a small cup of hot green tea at the end of a meal for all blood types. I'm calling it the emulsification that occurs between mastication and digestion. I can't exaggerate the benefits from a hot cup of green tea at the end of a meal. In myself, I'm finding less water retention and less thirst after a meal. It actually cleans my teeth at the end of a meal. Green tea can be used cold, also, either straight or mixed with some beneficial fruit juice. Green tea is considered beneficial due to its blood chemistry balancing and is also considered a cancer and diabetes superbeneficial as well. Just remember that any fruit juice used to mix with green tea can have large amounts of sugar added to them for flavor. Look at the ingredients and try to stay with natural sources and stay away from *all* sugar substitutes such as splenda, etc.

Horsetail is an herb that aids in calcium absorption and reduces inflammation. It can be taken as an extract or in capsule form. Avoid licorice at all costs; it increases blood pressure.

Milk Thistle could be a very beneficial herb to help in your chronic heartburn. Basically, milk thistle cleanses the liver thus causing an over-production of bile. Bile is the alkaline to the hydrochloric acid that is the acid in the stomach; the two tend to neutralize each other. In your case, your chronic heartburn could be the result of too much acid or not enough bile. Bile is produced by the liver and stored in the gall bladder, which secretes bile into the digestive tract near the duodenum, the first portion of the small intestines at the bottom of the stomach. Unabsorbed calcium can collect in the gall bladder and become gall stones, which can block the secretion of bile resulting in an acidic condition. Those without their gall bladders have to be careful taking milk thistle due to an over-production and automatic dumping of bile into the stomach resulting in an overall alkaline condition which causes nausea and vomiting. It's easily remedied if a few seedless grapes are eaten when nausea first begins. This is important because a short duration of milk thistle, the first one to two weeks, would be best for you. If your alkaline condition returns, the over-production of bile could cause some nausea. If this happens, eat a few seedless grapes and discontinue milk thistle. It's nothing dangerous; it's just that nausea sux.

Copper bracelets and copper jewelry change the skin color to green near the contact area due to the copper salts being absorbed through the skin and into the blood. In the blood, the copper ions attach loosely to the hemoglobin and inhibit inflammation throughout the body. While copper has scientific basis, magnets do not, yet. Maybe someday that research will find some basis for magnets, but as it is, not yet."

It could be said that her Addison's is being caused from a combination of too much folic acid from all the tomato products and not enough oils and nutrients from the lack of fish and vegetables. Is Addison's solely an A-type disease? How prevalent in other blood types? Has the adrenal cortex been damaged beyond repair or will a change in diet, and possibly exercise, bring it back?

Prostate Cancer In B-type Blood

Possible Equation:
B-type Adult Male + whole wheat + post nasal drip = Prostate Cancer

I have found a possible connection between sinusitis/rhinitis and prostate cancer. I have found that decades of continuous ingestion of whole wheat and whole wheat products in B-Type blood people causes the sinus to inflame causing an over-production of mucus. This could be caused from the ingestion of some natural chemical, such as lectins, in wheat itself that causes inflamed sinus or the resulting digestive imbalance occurring from the ingestion of wheat or a combination of both. Regardless, the resulting post-nasal drip inhibits proper gastric function and irritates the bowels causing more mucus production and more post-nasal drip and the cycle continues.

Over a period of years and even decades, the resulting imbalances in digestion and nutrients to the body cause glands to over-work and swell. They over-work because they have to perform the same function whether they have the proper nutrients to do the job or not. The prostate could become susceptible to malignant growths once this swelling / over-work got to the point where the body could not move malignant cells and waste away from the body fast enough. At the same time, the immunities are hampered by the ingestion of avoid foods, including whole wheat, and therefore can't readily adapt to ridding the body of toxins and poorly developed cells. At that point, a tumor could form.

Why is the prostate so susceptible to failure before anything else? Weakest link in the chain? It could be said that since the prostate is so close to a waste area, the urinary tract, and yet has to produce a substance, prostate fluid, that is foreign to something as acidic as uric acid, it could be overtly susceptible to increased infection-fighting activities throughout its life and therefore takes longer to recover from such attacks as infection and malignant cells. Who knows? I need much more data.

High cholesterol in A's & Anemia in O's

**Equations: A-type adult + meat = High Cholesterol
O-type adult - meat = Anemia**

One of the general conclusions drawn so far is O-type's who don't eat meat are anemic and A-type's who do eat meat have high cholesterol, as previously stated above. This has been an overwhelmingly consistent trend that I noticed only around the end of 2006. Therefore, finding anemia in A's and high cholesterol in O's has proven to be a challenge.

The chemistry here is easy to understand. O's have an acidic digestive tract while the A's have an alkaline system. The alkaline system doesn't breakdown the meats as well as the acidic system. Therefore, cholesterol, among other chemicals, do not get dissolved in the A digestive system and it piles up causing everything from atherosclerosis to COPD to virtually every cardio problem out there.

When I first noticed this trend about a year before this writing, I figured it would be easy to find an O-type with high cholesterol, if not an anemic A. However, it hasn't happened yet and I figure I just don't have enough information and/or I'm looking in the wrong place.

Can high cholesterol in A's be totally corrected by eliminating meat from their diets? So far, yes. More importantly, finding what would cause an O-type to have high cholesterol could spawn more questions and discoveries than we can possibly imagine at this point. Additionally, finding what would cause an A to be anemic could be a plethora of information that could lead in many unknown directions. I feel that this door of information will yield a tremendous amount of information in an immense area, when we open it.

Pork's Relationship To Tumors

Possible Equations:
O-type female + pork + venison = Benign breast tumors
A-type + pork + fish = Benign tumors

This is another trend that I have scant, little information. So far, I've noticed a slight trend with tumors and the ingestion of pork products. One poignant example is Susan (not her real name). A middle-aged, over-weight, O-type mother of three, Susan had malignant breast tumors in her thirties which were removed and she lived. At the time, pork products were big in her life. Her husband started deer hunting and venison made its way into her diet on a very regular basis for years. In her late forties she was diagnosed with breast tumors, but they were benign this time.

The theory is pork may have an amino acid profile that is too narrow to adequately supply the body with the proper variety of amino acids in their correct quantities. Of course, the body produces its own non-essential amino acids from the essential ones combined with resources from the body such as vitamins, enzymes and minerals. However, in creating the proper array of amino acids to properly rebuild cells, can the body run low or completely exhaust its supplies of resources to create and process those amino acids, thus creating an 'incomplete' cell that doesn't exactly function properly, but is so closely related to the properly built cell that the immunities, which are already hampered by a poor diet, don't recognize the cell as pathological and, therefore, allow it to continue to grow and reproduce? Is this a trend? Is this the basis for the creation of malignant tumors?

How To Use Conventional Medicine

**Possible Equation: O-type Adult Female + coffee =
Early and Difficult Menopause**

A Cure For Menopause

Diane (not her real name) started having hot flashes at age 39. Her mother went into early menopause in her late thirties and it continued for more than a decade, mostly due to the fact that her diet consisted mostly of foods that are listed as 'avoid' for her blood-type; she's an O-type. Diane had a lifetime of 'avoid' foods for her O-type blood, as well, before she found the blood-type diet.

Therefore, it was a true no-brainer to advise her to get her blood checked for low estrogen levels when the hot flashes started. I took her to a public testing facility and her blood test results confirmed an extremely low level of estrogen; almost zero.

She wanted to go to a doctor to have it all confirmed and see what can be done. Diane got the appointment, gave blood at the doctor's office and confirmed low estrogen levels in less than a month of continuing and worsening symptoms. The doctor gave the two classic choices given to all menopause patients: Wellbutrin for symptoms and birth control pills for estrogen replacement therapy. However, birth control pills for estrogen replacement therapy has such a risk of cancer that he said it would be best to wait and see how it goes with Wellbutrin before going to estrogen therapy. She would have to make a follow-up appointment.

The doctor gave her a prescription for Wellbutrin of which she immediately filled and started taking. It was effective for soothing mood swings, but all the other symptoms, including the hot flashes, were still present. However, after about a month, Wellbutrin's effectiveness waned to nothing. She started to wean herself off of Wellbutrin only to enter the horrible world of physical withdrawal. Wild mood swings, excessive depression and bizarre behavior ensued and only stayed in check due to her tremendous intellect. She had to notify human resources at her work to explain what was going on and why her work was suffering.

I told her to start a stabilizing combination of herbs which included mostly black cohosh. There are many products available and we chose one with a large amount of black cohosh. Additionally, she was advised to use progesterone crème, which provided balance; she was getting too much estrogen which was throwing off other levels.

These were difficult in keeping her levels correct due to the fact that her body simply wasn't producing estrogen, so it had nothing to work with. I started her drinking soy milk, which contains phytoestrogens and is a neutral food for her O-type blood. Lastly, Damiana, an herb that balances hormones and releases energy from the foods eaten, was the item that brought everything together. Not only did Damiana balance all the chemicals, but it soothed her mood swings dramatically. This also aided her physical withdrawal from Wellbutrin, as well.

So, basically, the soy milk provides phytoestrogens and the Damiana breaks apart the phytoestrogens into estrogen on the level that is safe and comfortable for the body. This is called estrogen replacement therapy done the natural, homeopathic way. Her hot flashes, which she was having about once every fifteen minutes, disappeared completely and never returned. Her mood went to steady, happy ambiance that doesn't change; no depression whatsoever.

To sum, conventional medicine, in this case, was not only ineffective, it was detrimental. The doctor has only two choices, mandated by the AMA and the insurance industry, when low estrogen levels are confirmed with blood tests: Wellbutrin for symptoms and birth control pills for estrogen replacement therapy. He never explained the waning effectiveness of Wellbutrin nor its physical withdrawal when stopping taking the drug due to its waning effectiveness. The doctor knows perfectly well that he can maximize his income by making sure the patient is unaware of the physical withdrawal of Wellbutrin, so the patient has to come back to the doctor for relief when things really go awry, thus charging for another doctor's appointment to the patient and the insurance company. Their only option left is a prescription for birth control pills for estrogen replacement that is such a carcinogen that even the doctor hesitated prescribing it, at first.

The only effective activity performed by the doctor, in this case, was providing a confirmation of the low estrogen levels in her blood that had already been confirmed by a publicly available testing facility. It's not a bad thing for a patient to use conventional medicine for diagnosis and second opinions, but it's completely another thing to use conventional medicine for treatment or for cure.

First of all, conventional medicine was built for treatment and was never intended for cure. If you notice, the only time conventional medicine aims for cure is when the disease is lethal. If the disease is not lethal, cure is never an option; only treatment is available, though there are generally cures available. However, if something can be cured, then continuing treatment is no longer an option and the flow of money ceases. It's a very old and a very simple story: the business of medicine.

Lastly, the bottom line is conventional medicine is most useful for diagnosis and second opinions. Prescriptions can be written, but they don't always have to be filled. Conventional drugs should be relegated to the last option and never seen as the first option, unless there are no other options, which is possible, but rare. Sometimes conventional medicines and homeopathic medicines have to be used together, as in the case of anti-biotics and pro-biotics; anti-biotics to kill the infection and pro-biotics to replace the beneficial bacteria in the lower colon that was killed by the side-effects of the anti-biotic. Education is the key to health.

A Sore Back Story

It seems the back is the most prolific source of complaints of Homo sapiens. It should be no surprise. After all, we walk and stand upright. The erector spinae is always in an isometric position; throughout the day, erector spinae is tense but not moving and in a near-stretched position. Therefore, when it gets sore, stretching provides little relief. It gets sore because it's weak. It's as simple as that. Given a strong, well-exercised erector spinae, the person can sit in one position all day, every day without issue as long as that person continues to keep it strong with regular, consistent exercise.

Once injured, the back is almost impossible to bring back to normal. There are always some lingering effects of the injury throughout life. Exercise and blood-type diet aids with the injured back as it does with the non-injury. It's just that if the back, or any part of the body, is preserved, it will continue to function without fail. Keeping everything preserved is our life's job.

A client came to me with complaints of a sore back. She was middle-aged with several kids in their young adolescence. She was very busy. She came daily to the gym at which I was working and kept a very regular and consistent exercise routine. However, this sore back had just come up over the previous 4 to 6 months. There were no previous injuries and no lapses in exercise routine.

Therefore, I gave her an exercise to do that is used for the true beginner or the geriatric. Though I knew she was no beginner or geriatric, I knew we had to start at the beginning to be sure we could do the harder stuff. Additionally, the exercise I started her with I call the 'superman': an isometric for the erector spinae that puts the client on the floor in the flying superman position lifting hands and feet while leaving the stomach pressed against the floor. She was to do this for a count of five and then relax, repeating ten times or until pain.

She did this for about a week and she came back to me saying that it helped, but the pain would return every time. I told her at that point, before we can do anything else, she would need to go to an orthopedic for at least an x-ray, if not more, to rule out anything that would be causing this pain other than simply weak muscles, which seemed unlikely to me right from the beginning just because she was already active in the gym for years with no problem.

She didn't like that idea. She pestered me for weeks for more and different back exercises so she could continue building it up. I obstinately refused. I repeatedly told her that I would be more than happy to help her once we got the OK from the orthopedic, but not before under any circumstances. She could have gone to another trainer, but she said she wanted to stay with me.

The weeks went by and she disappeared. I forgot about her and I left the gym at which I was working for brighter horizons. About a year later, I was walking through the grocery store with a friend when this lady came up to me all flustered and very happy to see me. She exclaimed she was so happy she had found me to tell me her story.

Basically, she took my advice and made an appointment with an orthopedic. The doctor took an x-ray and found a cyst growing on her spinal cord. It had started to wind its way into the spinal cord, but she caught it early, before it actually entered into the nerves themselves. Had she waited much longer, she would have been paralyzed or dead. The doctor operated and she recovered with no issues. She went on to bigger and better back exercises.

The moral of this story is that there are many conditions that require conventional medicine all the way to fruition. Generally, those examples require surgery, but not always. In this case, a second opinion wasn't necessary; the cyst was easy to see in the x-ray, surgery is the only way to get rid of it and speed was of the essence. Many people would try ridding her cyst with diet, but that would have been disastrous. Such conditions as cysts, tumors, warts and other growths may be prevented with diet and exercise, but once present, conventional medicine is essential before they spread, possibly including surgical removal.

Longevity, especially in A's

I have found how a smoker lives to be 101 years old. He has A Type blood and eats fish & rice on a daily basis. I have found entire Polynesian A-type families who regularly smoke, eat rice and fish and live into their third digits.

The Wish List

February 2008

—O-Type blood with high cholesterol.
—Athletic O's with diabetes and sedentary O's with arthritis.
—A-Types with acid indigestion, heartburn.
—Mothers' Blood Types.
—Romantic couples who have been together for at least twenty years.
—Blood-types by occupation.
—Centurions.

—**O-Type blood with high cholesterol.** So far, as of January 29, 2008, all of the high cholesterol clients have turned out to have A-type blood. I have yet to find an O with high cholesterol. Since A's have an alkaline digestive tract and O's have the acidic one, meat eaten by A's may not break down the LDL fully and it would collect in the arteries giving an elevated cholesterol reading.

Therefore, I'm looking for O-type's with high cholesterol. In trying to find this supposed anomaly, the collected statistics should prove or disprove the overall trend.

—**Athletic O's with diabetes and sedentary O's with arthritis.** We already know that white potatoes and O-type blood agglutinate improperly settling in the joints to become arthritis later. I have found two types of O's: arthritic and diabetic. What is so striking is they are totally exclusive; that is, if one O is arthritic, diabetes is never an issue whereas an O with diabetes never seems to get arthritis.

Furthermore, it's starting to look like physically active O's are the arthritic O's whereas the diabetic O's are sedentary. It could be said that the active O, who is inflaming the joints, ligaments, muscles, etc. as a normal reaction of exercise, is also burning the excess glucose in the blood thus leaving the pancreas to work less. Arthritis is the result instead of diabetes.

On the other hand, the sedentary O never inflames anything by not exercising. The glucose levels don't get burned off by exercise. Instead, the glucose levels have to be chemically altered with insulin and stored as fat, which is the job of the pancreas. The pancreas eventually burns-out and ceases producing enough insulin to properly keep glucose levels in the blood. Diabetes results instead of arthritis.

Therefore, as of January 29, 2008, I'm looking for the athletic O with diabetic tendencies, or actual diagnosis, and the sedentary O with arthritis. In trying to find these supposed anomalies, this traditional theory of sedentary and active O's may be backed up by overwhelming numbers; or disproved completely.

—A-Types with acid indigestion, heartburn. A's have an alkaline digestive tract and never complain of heartburn. I have found the only A's who complain of heartburn have Addison's disease and complain also of a craving for salt, a known symptom of Addison's. They habitually eat tomato products extensively, eat very little vegetables and almost never eat fish.

Addison's disease can be caused by the immunities attacking the outer layer of the adrenal gland known as the adrenal cortex. This autoimmune action could be precipitated by a bad diet causing the antigens to falsely agglutinate to improper tissues as a result of the chemicals from the avoid foods for A-type blood. These chemicals, such as an overdose of folic acid imbalanced with a deficit of all the nutrients from essential fish and vegetables, could cause the auto-immunities to attack such tissues as the adrenal cortex, not to mention other places.

The problem with Addison's disease is the fact that it leads to an entire host of classic diseases including diabetes. It could be the bottleneck to a number of ailments that could be easily avoided.

Therefore, as of January 29, 2008, I am looking for people with A-type blood who complain of heartburn. In trying to find this anomaly, the Addison connection to A's could be proven or disproved and thusly prove or disprove the bottleneck that could be the source of disease for 40% of the world's population.

—Mothers' Blood Types. I've found some consistent trends that seem to follow the mitochondrial DNA passed down maternally. These trends have the potential of sub-dividing the species, homo sapiens, into 16 to 64 different sub-species.

As of February 4, 2008, there is far too little data to even know how many sub-species there are. If it differs by blood group, then we'll have 16, but if it differs by genetic ties to RH factors, then there could be as many as 64.

As a note, recently I have found a possibility that may suggest there are only 16, rather thand 64, which I had been starting to lean towards. The bottom line is I need large statistics to prove or disprove these trends.

—Romantic couples who have been together for at least twenty years. In my research, I started to notice that married couples who had been married for decades had a high percentage of common blood types; that is, they were pairs of the same blood types whether it be a pair of O's or a pair of A's, or a pair of B's. I don't have enough AB's in my data to establish a trend, yet, but I need all types.

—Blood-types by occupation. In my research, I have found a disproportionate number of B-types in I.T. departments; computer geeks. In general, B-types represent approximately 12% of the population, whereas I have found I.T. departments are populated with over half having B-type blood. I know of one small I.T. Department that, so far, has 100% B-type blood.

It just so happens that people with B-type blood are statistically more susceptible to nerve disorders, such as ALS. Is there a connection? Do blood-types naturally gravitate to certain professions?

Before any of that can even gets close to an answer, the overall trend has to be confirmed with large numbers. Therefore, I need occupations listed by blood types; that is, workers and their blood-types in mass quantities.

—Centurions. In the research, I stumbled upon entire Polynesian A-type families who regularly smoke, eat rice and fish and live into their third digits. This seems to be how a smoker lives to be 100 years old. He has A Type blood and eats fish & rice on a daily basis.

Obviously, this needs big statistics to be proven at the very least. I need centurions listed by blood-types.

Possible Equation: A-type + fish + rice = Longevity

Selected Sample Data

Male—O type—Born in 1991. Exercises once per week on average. Non-smoker. At age 14, he is starting to feel the effects of early hypoglycemia. He has been found to be in highest percentile for developing diabetes as tested by PANDA Research Group; a pediatric genetic research facility for diabetes. As of September, he added potatoes (french fries) back in his diet, somewhat, and has morning energy issues frequently.

Male—B Type—Born in 1994. No exercise. Non-smoker. No symptoms; probably too young. He is not following the B-Type diet.

Male—B Type—Born in 1988. No exercise. Non-smoker. He is overweight by about 20 lbs. Started the B-Type diet in mid-July and stuck about 95% strictly out of avoids and about 80% in beneficial foods. He lost 10 lbs in 10 days with no exercise whatsoever. Two weeks into it, school started and he is routinely eating irregularly. He has been told that this should put his body into the starvation mode and he will gain weight dramatically if he continues; he did better. As of August 12, 2005, he is avoiding approx. 70%, benefiting rarely (below 20%), has lost 11 lbs and approx. 2 inches around his waist. He is still urinating more. He has started a cardio routine 3 days a week consisting of 30 minutes of circuit training. As of September 20, 2005, he has lost 15 lbs. and approximately 2½ inches around his waist. As of October 4, 2005, he had started circuit training last month and, as a result, he has gained 5 lbs of muscle and his waist has remained at 2 ½ inches lost, so far.

Female—A Type—Born in 1961. Non-smoker. Little to no exercise only in the past year. No exercise before that. Has had Crohn's disease to the point of surgery in her twenties. Severe depression runs in her and her brother, but not noticeable in her parents. Her brother committed suicide in the early 1980's due to depression when he was approximately 18 years old. She is benefiting and avoiding at 0%. She wrote on August 12, 2005, "There is no way I can be a vegetarian. I don't eat a lot of beef and pork but I do eat a fair amount of chicken. I do fairly well eating a lot of vegetables but I CANNOT be reading labels on foods and being sure I only eat certain things. Just not in my make up." In mid 2005, she started having night sweats of which her hormones checked OK. PAP smear was OK. In 2006, she started reading labels and is doing much better.

Male—A Type—Born in 1961. No exercise. Smoker since high school. He was overweight by about 30 lbs with most of it on his waist. His diet was very poor for an A-type before the A-type diet. His mother is an A-type. He started the A-Type diet on July 23, 2005 at 185 pounds. He is avoiding at almost 100% and benefiting at about 85%. In the first ten days, he lost 10 lbs. He has experienced increased urination and increased defecation; one day he took 5 craps. At the 3-week mark, he has lost almost 15 lbs and has moved his belt down two notches. At the one-month mark, he has lost 21 pounds at 164 pounds, his pants are falling off of him and his belt is down almost three notches. His boss remarked that his neck and face appear smaller. He was wondering if he was doing cocaine or something. As of November 25, 2005, he has lost almost 30 pounds.

Male—A Type—Born in 1965. No exercise. Non-smoker. Overweight by about 40 lbs with most of it on his waist. Auto mechanic and always on the go; very active work environment. Started the A-Type diet at the beginning of August, 2005. In one week, he lost 7 lbs and one notch on his belt. He has experienced increased urination and increased defecation; everything OK. By August 20, 2005, he reports his servings at meals are smaller. Instead of getting 2 and 3 large servings, he feels full after only one small serving. Additionally, he says the single small serving tends to last at least a third longer than his past large multiple servings after any one meal. His sugar cravings are gone. He says he use to reach for snacks all the time at work. Now, he simply never thinks about it; it never occurs to him. His hunger pangs are much less severe when they happen which are far less frequent than before the A Type diet. Urination and defecation have tapered to near normal. He lost a total of 20 lbs. Approximately a month later, he quit the diet and went back to a poor A-type diet. As of November 1, 2006, he has put back all the weight plus, at least, 25% more. He is at the largest size he has ever been in his life.

Male—B Type—Born in 1918. Died in 2003. Non-smoker. Light calisthenics with light weights regularly every morning. Avid tennis player from late sixties to 2000. Golfer from the 1950's to 2002. Basketball in high school and after. When he was a kid he ate small game such as rabbit regularly. By the late 1960's, he changed to shredded wheat every morning and chicken many times a week, which both have highly detrimental lectins to B-Types, yet wondered why his waist was always blowing up and his nose was always running. This went on for decades before he died. He actually started eating that way when, in the late sixties, he was diagnosed as diabetic, mostly due to his lack of exercise and poor diet which at the time included daily milkshakes and fast food. Since he knew that diabetes "ran" in his family, he changed his diet and started playing tennis heavily. He turned it around and successfully kept it from going into full-blown diabetes for the rest of his life. Prostate cancer was diagnosed in 1991 and the prostate was removed. In 2002, bone cancer, which had metastisized from the prostate cancer, was discovered in his L5 vertebra and was later to be determined to be widespread throughout his body. It would appear he swapped diabetes for cancer.

Male—AB Type—Born in 1987. Lanky body type. No exercise. Non-smoker. Acne present over entire body and face. Avoiding 0% and benefiting 0%.

Female—O Type—Born in 1965—No exercise. Smoker since mid-teens. Woefully underweight. Mother is an O-type. Father died in late fifties from a heart attack. Diagnosed diabetic and hypothyroidism in 2004 and later that year became full-blown diabetic needle-pusher. Dairy was a staple throughout life with her and her sisters and they would drink it like water, which they do to this day. The four players are the mother and the three sisters, daughter1, daughter2 and daughter3, born in that order. The mother, daughter1 and daughter3 are all needle-pushing diabetics. Daughter2, the middle daughter and the only one who moved away permanently when she was 18 at college never to return again, never developed the disease. She moved in with her staunchly Italian husband's family and never left. Her diet changed dramatically at age 18 and never went back. I think it's a little more than just ironic that daughter2 didn't develop diabetes when everyone else in her family, past and present, did develop the disease, while at the same time she just happens to be the only one in the family who dramatically changed her diet which has remained the same for the past 25 years. At the very least, it could be said that genetics play a much smaller role than what we had all figured, including me.

Male—O Type—Born in 1962—No exercise. Smoker since college. Approx. 25 lbs overweight. Sedentary desk job. Family history of colon issues. Eats very little dairy overall. As of August 13, 2005, he is benefitting very little and avoiding at about 40%. Yet, he says he has lost about 5 lbs. As of August 29,

2005, he is benefiting more, about 40%, and avoiding well, at about 90%, yet he has lost 10 lbs. with no exercise.

Female—O Type—Born in 1971?—No exercise. Non-smoker. Approx. 25 lbs overweight. Drinks milk like water. As of August 13, 2005, she is having a very difficult time restricting the dairy and has made no progress elsewhere.

Female—O Type—Born in 1970—Non-smoker. Significant health issues: anorexic & bulimic 1988 to 2002, OCD, alcoholic, septic shock surgery in 2002, abdominal hernia surgery in 2004, gall bladder removed in 2004, severe pancreatitis 2004 through 2005. In 1988, she moved in with her grandmother and started eating wheat germ on a daily basis, which happens to be the same time her ED (eating disorder) started. For a year, 1991 and 1992, while she was heavily into anorexia, she ate wheat pretzels with much mustard, one jar of pickles, baked potatoes with much ketchup and nothing else on a daily basis; all avoids for an O. Bulimia started in late 1992; she kept only broccoli and green beans and vomited everything else. As of July, 2005, she is doing no exercise. However, she was religiously exercising up to 2004, but quit due to symptoms due to alcoholism and crystal meth dependency. As of August, 2005, she's been eating McDonald's grilled chicken sandwich's, hoagie's, no breakfasts, dinners were generally chicken. In October 2005, she got religion in a big way. It appears to have helped to get her away from the alcohol. As of December 7, 2005, she says she has not had a drink for over a month. Her diet consists of mostly red meat such as hamburger since about October. At this point she has started to get her life back on track; difficult to know whether it's religion, diet or the combination.

Female—A Type—Born in 1964—No exercise. Smoker. Recovered anorexic. At the height of her anorexia in the early 1990's, she ate nothing, but salad, canned vegetables—green beans, carrots. When her energy would get very low, she would eat a piece of bread or something small and starchy.

Male—B Type—Born in 1964?—No exercise. Non-smoker. Sedentary job. Drinks liquor and beer every night after work just to relax; not to the point of interfering with his job. As of August, 2005, he says he can't follow the B Type diet and is currently not following any guidelines.

Female—A Type—Born in 1961. Smoker. No exercise. Woefully underweight by at least 15 lbs. Very high strung; weight fluctuates with stress. Extremely poor diet; eats whenever hungry, but eats simple sugars, complex sugars, intermittent sources of protein, virtually no vegetables and drinks whole milk like water; except milk, all in small quantities. Family history is picture-perfect with disease-free longevity. Had cervical cancer in 1997 of which surgery solved completely. However, as of 2004, she started chronic vaginal bleeding and slight hot flashes. Doctors have found her thyroid functioning properly and no sign of diabetes. PAP smear is OK. As of August 2005, her hormones have not been checked and she says there's no way she can do the A type diet. Her vaginal bleeding stopped. As of mid-November, 2005, her blood profile came back with cholesterol at 242 with her LDL at 160. I've noticed a grey-ish complexion.

Female—A Type—Born in 1971—Non-Smoker. No exercise. She says she's a vegetarian, but she's eating many avoid foods for A-Type diet, not getting any protein to speak of and refuses to eat any fish whatsoever. Her diet includes large amounts of diet soda daily. As of August, 2005, she has extensive acne in the face but nowhere else on her body. She suffers from headaches and can't sleep well.

Male—O Type—Born in 1965? Non-Smoker. No exercise. He is approximately 20 lbs overweight. He has been following the O Type diet at about 70% and never knew it. His diet had to be adjusted minimally to stay clearly on the O-Type diet.

Male—O Type—Born in 1974. Non-Smoker; quit in 1998, smoked for three years while deployed in middle east. Exercises 3 times a week; 45 minutes of aerobics. He says he's not in good shape. He used to be very athletic back in 2001; used to eat over 5000 calories per day and train heavily twice a day; running more than 25 miles per week; weighed 175 at the time. Not overweight now; 185 lbs. 5' 11". In a 24-hour period in September 2005, he ate bagel, peanut butter, coffee, salmon, roasted red potatoes, salad, breast of chicken and couscous. He suffers from heartburn to the extreme. Arthritis runs on Mother's side.

Male—A Type—Born in 1962. Non-smoker. No exercise. He is approximately 15 lbs underweight. Alcoholic to the extreme; drinks liquor throughout the day, every day. Has a history of crystal meth which has increased his need for liquor just to get to sleep, though his consumption of liquor throughout the years never really went below drinking throughout each day. His father died of pancreatitis as a direct result of alcohol, though he was never an alcoholic, in that it never interfered with his life, i.e. job, wife, family, etc. His mother died of lung cancer and was a heavy smoker for decades. His diet stays mostly in the avoid section for A type blood.

Female—A Type. Born in 1970's. Non-smoker. Exercises regularly at Bally's in the mornings. Mother of three children. Born with hole in heart and had open heart surgery as a child. No complications to present. Remarkably, there is absolutely no cancer in her family history which goes back several generations on both sides, which have a great deal of longevity on both. The only exception in her family tree was a distant relative who died of a heart attack in his mid-fifties. Diagnosed with multiple sclerosis in 2000; currently taking medications to help with symptoms which are unnoticeable. I told her that MS is one of the most mis-diagnosed diseases. Though she is an A, she appears to be hitting her beneficials and neutrals much more than most A-Type blood people. She eats very little meats. Not a big fan of fish. Cheese (blue cheese) is a weakness for her, but not too bad. She doesn't drink milk. She loves peanuts and peanut butter. Wheat (English muffins) is a weakness. She's big into vegetables (onions, garlic). Honeydew is a weakness for her, as is soda.

Female—O Type. Born in 1972. Non-smoker. No exercise. Mother of three small children. Eats no dairy. She craves rice and eats a lot of it. Eats mostly vegetables. One day's staple diet: egg, half a small bagel, rice, ground beef. No medications, no medical conditions. High blood pressure, arthritis runs in family. Mother has hemorrhoids.

Female—O Type—Born in 1968. Smoker; one pack per day. Non-drinker. No exercise. Asthmatic. Fiber cystic breast disease diagnosed in 1991; no complications other than pain during PMS. Scrambled eggs, toast, Dad born in 1946; no health problems; smoked for decades and quit in 2000. Mother (O-Type) born in 1948; always in bad health; asthma, emphasema, lordosis, arthritis, non-drinker, non-smoker. While the client was pregnant, she ate extreme amounts of snickers bars, gained 80 lbs and yet never even came close to gestational diabetes nor diabetes later in life.

Male—O Type—Born in mid-70's. Non-smoker. Non-drinker. No exercise. He has to adjust diet slightly to be on target. However, those slight things to be changed are very difficult because they have become a daily cycle. As of

November, 2005, he drinks coffee during the day to stay awake at a sedentary IT job. At night he can't get to sleep because of the coffee all day, so he eats ice cream which makes him drowsy and he sleeps. The next day he's sluggish because of the ice cream the night before and so he drinks coffee to make it through the day and the cycle continues.

Female—A Type—Born in mid-70's. Non-smoker. Non-drinker. Exercises five days a week. She eats surprisingly close to a beneficial A-type diet eating what her body calls for, just like an O-type. Her mother is an O type.

Male—A Type—Born in 1962. Survived heart attack in 2000. Very poor A-type diet before finding the A-type diet, which he started in November of 2005.

Female (Nurse)—AB Type—Born in 1956. Breast cancer runs in her family. Her son is not an AB nor is her mother. (However, information is scant due to an uncooperative attitude from her. She was very distrustful and not ready to give information. She's the only entry in the data who was pushed to give information solely because her blood type is so rare and information on AB's is difficult and rare to obtain.)

Male (waiter)—A Type—Philippine. Born in 1973. Smoker. No exercise. Staple diet is mainly chicken, fish, rice and no breakfast. Not much beef or dairy in diet. His grandfather, A Type, was a smoker, ate mostly fish & rice his entire life and died at 101 of pneumonia not long after quitting smoking which he had done for the majority of his life. His grandmother, A Type, as of December 2005, was 99 years old and had just recently started to quit smoking due to failing health. Both grandparents and the rest of his family are in the Philippines. There has never been any sign of cancer in their known family history and it's a large family that keeps rice & fish as a daily staple diet for their lives in the Philippines.

Female (waitress)—O Type—Philippine. Born in 1984. Social drinker (2 limit). Eats rib-eye's. No heartburn.

Male—A Type—Born in 1938. Weighs 280 lbs. 6' 3". Non-smoker. Non-drinker since 1990. In a 24-hour period in December, 2005, he ate ice cream, milk shake, ribs, salad, chicken, Pollock, sausage, jalapeño poppers, pumpkin pie, apple cobbler for lunch, slice of bread with peanut butter for breakfast, meat loaf, mashed potatoes, gravy, corn, roll for dinner, eggs for dinner. High blood pressure; on medication. Peripheral neuropathy is his feet; really bad feet. Circulation is bad in feet; hammer toes. Bad back. Sleep apnea. Diagnosed as diabetic in 2007.

Male—O Type—Born in late 1960's. (2007) High blood pressure; on medication. Eats pistachios at night before bedtime; suggested walnuts as an alternative. Found blood-type and this diet in March, 2007, and is adjusting his diet. He was avoiding meat as much as possible due to societal dogma. Stopped Milk, pistachios, reduced coffee intake. Bread, ice cream and coffee are still issues. Vanilla soy milk instead of milk. No milk equals no allergies. Cereal and milk at night was making him have "blah" days; years ago he stopped drinking alcohol in an attempt to stop the "blah" days which alleviated it to a degree but he still had them; once he stopped the cereal and milk at night, his "blah" days disappeared immediately and totally, virtually overnight.

Female—A Type—Born in 1963. (2007) Exercises by walking seven days a week and weight-bearing exercise once or twice a week. Diet is very poor; never eats a balanced meal; always grabbing small snacks (pretzels, tofu) throughout the day; cooks for kids and husband, but never eats the meal (not ED). The only good part of her diet is the sushi she eats once or twice a week. Other than bad knees from incorrect exercising in the gym, hot-and-cold temperatures on the body, reminiscent of the start of menopause, is the only other symptom she has, which she says she has always had throughout her life.